# Clean Food

By

## Rayan Parker

# Table of Contents

# Introduction

Did you know that the food choices you make every day affects your health? The quality of food you eat can affect how you feel today, tomorrow and also in the future. If you fail to deliberately choose healthy foods now, then you may experience the effects of either making the wrong choices or leaving your health to chance.

Interestingly, good nutrition is an essential aspect of leading a healthy lifestyle and when combined with exercise, adequate water, sleep and others, you will be able to maintain a healthy weight. It will also help you to promote your overall health while reducing your risk of chronic diseases such as cancer and heart disease. What are the best kinds of food that are suitable for your health? How can you ensure that you eat healthy foods and live a healthy lifestyle?

This content will focus on nutrition ideas, the importance of fruits, vegetables, sleep, water and living a healthy lifestyle. By embracing the right nutrition, you will not only increase your level of energy but will improve your health significantly and prevent most diseases which are often caused by unhealthy lifestyles and consumption of junk and processed foods. Understand that the content in this book is meant to serve as information and does not in any way replace the advice of a medical professional.

Are you always confused and overwhelmed by the different views of nutrition experts out there on the internet? Do you find most diet advice you see online conflicting and so complicated that you stand no chance of implementing them successfully? The right diet and nutrition for you does not have to be complicated and that's what this book is all about – simple and easy ideas on the best choices when it comes to nutrition. Are you ready to discover the truth? Let's begin!

# Chapter One
# Healthy Eating

Generally, people tend to believe that eating a healthy diet has to do with so many restrictions, deprivations of the kind of foods you love, strict limitations and even staying unrealistically thin. Well, that's not what a healthy diet is all about; it has to do with feeling great, eating to improve your health, having more energy and giving your mood a boost.

The focus of this chapter is on healthy eating which is not unnecessarily complicated. Are you feeling so overwhelmed by the number of conflicting nutrition and diet advice all over the internet? Well, the good news is that you're not alone! Interestingly, when you go online in search of the best advice on the kind of healthy diet to eat, for every expert you meet that informs you that a particular kind of food is the best for you, you are likely going to meet another expert telling you the opposite.

This throws you into serious confusion right; who's telling the truth? You even find yourself in serious analysis paralysis and may just resolve to eat whatever comes your way. Truthfully, some kinds of food or nutrients have proved over time to have beneficial effects on mood and your health, but your overall dietary pattern is most crucial.

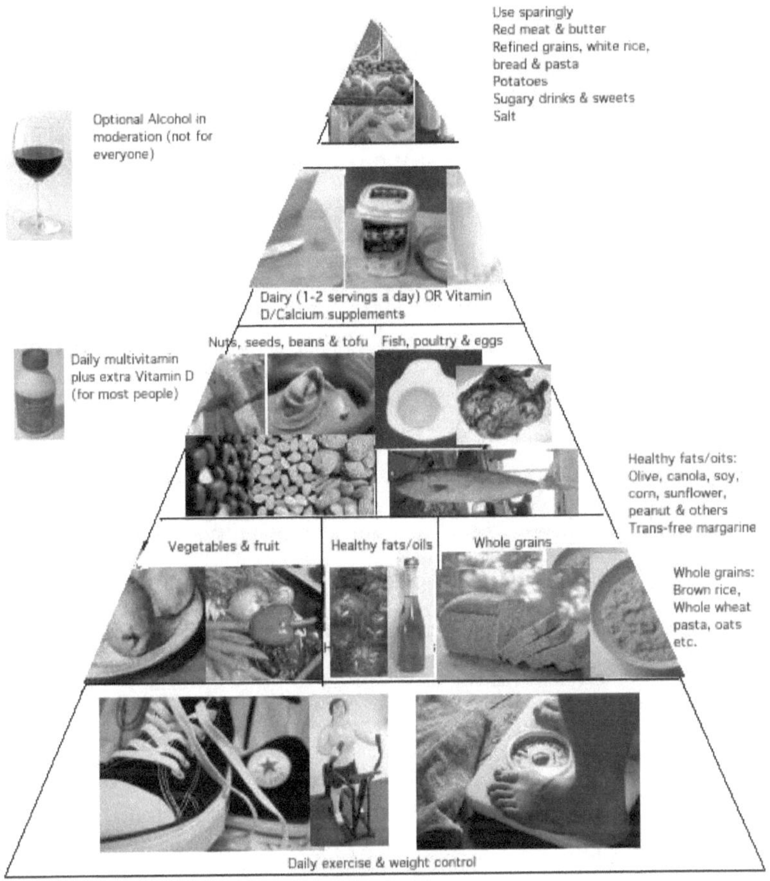


Understand that the foundation of a healthy diet is to replace all processed food with real food. You can positively transform the way you feel, think and look by simply eating foods that are as close as possible to how nature made them. My goal is to eliminate the confusion out there and provide simple ways to create (and stick to) a tasty nutritious and varied diet which will not only be good for your body but also your mind.

So, we begin by taking a look at the Harvard eating pyramid which contains straightforward information about the kind of foods and activities you need to stay healthy, energized and productive.

When you take a look at the Harvard Eating Pyramid which represents the latest nutritional science, you will find the best foods for your body. The widest part of the pyramid found at the bottom represents the things that are most important while the ones at the narrow top are the ones you need to eat sparingly – if at all. Does this make any sense? All through this book, we shall be going through some of these items so watch out.

## The Fundamentals of Healthy Eating - Essential Nutrients

Nutrition is regarded as the consumption of food which is considered in relation to our body's dietary needs. So, poor nutrition may likely lead to increased susceptibility to disease, reduced immunity, reduced productivity, and impaired physical and mental development. Good nutrition, on the other hand, refers to an adequate, well-balanced diet which is combined with regular physical activity and this is essential to good health.

A healthy diet involves the preparation of the food as well as the storage methods, which helps to preserve the nutrients from oxidation, heat or leaching and also lower the risk of food-borne illnesses. The consumption of healthy nutritious diet has repeatedly shown to prevent several diseases such as cancer. Undoubtedly, good nutrition is essential to the prevention of diseases; it's vital to good health and essential for healthy growth and development not only for kids but also for adults.

Actually, some extreme diets may tend to suggest otherwise, but the truth is that every one of us needs a good balance of fat, fiber, protein, vitamins, minerals and carbohydrates in our diets to sustain a healthy body. Rather than eliminate certain categories of food from your diet, the best option is to choose the healthiest options from each category.

Regardless of the opinion of nutrition experts, one thing is certain; they all agree that we need the essential nutrients. However, some may differ on the right quantity that we need to eat to stay healthy. So, let's take a look at some of these essential nutrients, what they do in our body system and how we can get them. You may be wondering what essential nutrients are. They are compounds that our body can't make and even if our body makes them, the quantity produced isn't sufficient for us.

According to the World Health Organization (WHO), these essential nutrients need to come from the food we eat and they're crucial for the prevention of diseases, for good health and growth. Generally, there are many essential nutrients; however, they are classified into two main categories – micronutrients and macronutrients. Some good examples of micronutrient include minerals and vitamins and our body can strive with small doses of these nutrients.

On the other hand, macronutrients are eaten in large amounts. They include the primary building blocks of our diet which provide us with energy – fat, protein and carbohydrates. Let's go through some of these essential nutrients.

**Protein**

The primary reason why protein is very popular, especially in the workout community is that it is essential for good health. It actually provides the building blocks of the body; in fact, all the cells in our body from the skin, to hair, to the bone contains protein. Interestingly, 16 percent of the weight of the body of an average person is composed of protein.

Unless necessary (through ketosis), protein is not always used to fuel the body. They are made up of various amino acids and even though our body is capable of creating amino acids on its own, there are some that we can only get from the food we eat. Our body requires a variety of amino acids for it to function properly.

There are several sources of protein, but in line with our goal, we shall point out the healthy sources. Apart from popular sources of protein such as fish, meat, and eggs, there are also other plant-based sources of protein like soy, beans, nuts and various kinds of grain. The quantity of protein you need each day depends on several factors like your age and how active you are.

**Carbohydrates**

Well, one of the most popular diets out there is the low carb diet for weight loss. But you shouldn't allow this to fool you. As earlier mentioned, you need all these essential nutrients in moderate amounts. According to Mayo Clinic, carbohydrates are crucial for a healthy body; they help to fuel the body and protect it against diseases. They should comprise 45 to 65 percent of your total daily calories.

Understand that the type of carbohydrate you eat matters significantly – some are healthier than the others. So, it's better to go for the healthier ones like beans, whole grains, fruits and fiber-rich vegetables instead of products with added sugar and refined grains.

**Fats**

Generally, in the food and nutrition sector, fats often get a bad reputation; however, this isn't very correct. Based on recent studies, it's clear that healthy fats are a crucial aspect of a healthy diet. In fact, the Harvard Medical School disclosed that it supports several functions of the body like blood clotting, building cells, vitamin and mineral absorption and muscle movement.

Although fat is quite high in calories, those calories are a vital source of energy for the body. The World Health Organization recommends that our daily calories, which come from fat should be under 30 percent. When you increase your intake of healthy fats, it can help you to decrease your risk of heart disease and type II diabetes, properly balance your blood sugar and increase your brain function. Also, healthy fats are powerful anti-inflammatories and are capable of lowering your risk of cancer, Alzheimer's disease and arthritis.

What are the healthy sources of fats? Actually, omega-3 and omega-6 fatty acids are the most popular unsaturated fats. The unsaturated fats are vital for your body. The reason is that the essential fatty acids that they provide can't be produced by your body. Some healthy sources of these fats include fish, nuts, vegetable oils (such as avocado, flaxseed, and olive), and seeds.

You can also get plant-based fats in the form of medium-chain triglycerides from coconut oil. This provides significant health benefits such as appetite control and faster utilization by organs as fuel. As much as possible, you need to avoid Trans fats and also reduce the quantity of saturated animal-based fats such as red meat, ice cream, cheese and butter.

**Vitamins**

One of the key benefits of vitamins is that they help to ward off diseases and keep us healthy. Also, our body requires these micronutrients to empower its functions. Generally, we have 13 essential vitamins required by our body to function properly and this includes vitamins A, C, B6, and D. Every single type of vitamin plays a vital role in our body and not having sufficient amount of these vitamins can lead to various health issues and diseases.

If you need a healthy skin, bones and vision, then you need vitamins. They help to lower the risk of lung and prostate cancer and are strong antioxidants. You're not likely going to need vitamin supplements if you eat a varied and properly balanced diet which comprises fruits and vegetables with a normal and healthy functioning digestive tract.

## Minerals

Just like vitamins, minerals also support our body. They are essential for various body functions like the regulation of your metabolism, helping you stay properly hydrated, and building of strong bones and teeth. Among the most common types of minerals include calcium, zinc and iron.

Apart from helping to strengthen the bones, calcium which is a mineral helps in maintaining a healthy blood pressure, nerve signal transmission and muscle contraction and relaxation. On the other hand, zinc boosts our immune system and wound healing, while iron supports red blood cells and hormone creation.

## Water

Although we shall be taking a deeper look at the importance of water, it's important to know that about 62 percent of our body weight is water. It's possible for you to go for weeks without food and still survive. But you may not be able to last for a few days without water. It's necessary for every system in our body; it helps to improve your brain function and mood. Water also serves as a shock absorber as well as a lubricant.

## Phytochemicals

The effect some trace chemicals (known as phytochemicals) have upon human health is attracting more interests recently. Most of these nutrients are often found in edible plants, especially the colorful fruits and vegetables as well as other organisms such as fungi, algae and seafood.

The impact of phytochemicals increasingly survive severe testing by key health organizations. Among the principal classes of phytochemicals are polyphenol antioxidants. These are chemicals known to provide several health benefits to the cardiovascular system as well as the immune system – chemicals that are known to down-regulate the formation of "reactive oxygen species" and these are the main chemicals in cardiovascular disease.

# Chapter Two

# Adding Fruits & Vegetables to Your Diet

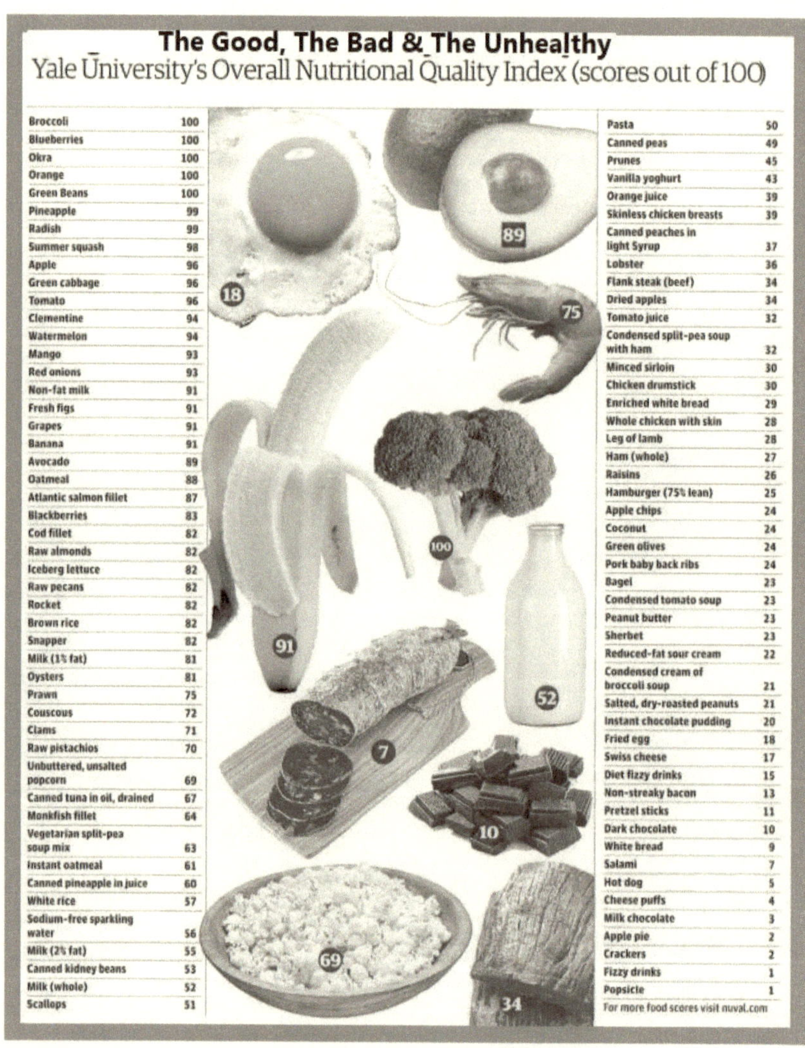



Having established the foundation of every healthy diet, let's take it a step further by going through the best kind of foods you need to eat. Take a good look at the food chart above; you will discover that the foods with the highest scores are fruits and vegetables. Most of the ones with the lower scores are processed foods. In fact, fizzy drinks and Popsicle occupy the bottom position with a score of one while top on the chart are vegetables and fruits such as orange, blueberries, okra, green beans and broccoli.

Did you know that a diet which is rich in fruits and vegetables can help lower the risk of heart disease and stroke, lower blood pressure, prevent some types of cancer, have a positive effect upon blood sugar (this helps to control your appetite), and lower the risk of eye and digestive problems? In fact, you can make gains in your weight loss efforts by eating non-starchy vegetables and fruits such as pears, green leafy vegetables, and apples.

They can help to prevent blood sugar spikes, which often increases hunger because of their low glycemic loads. There are at least nine different families of fruits and vegetables and each one of them has hundreds of different plant compound that provide several health benefits. You can give your body the mix of nutrients it requires by eating a variety of types and colors of fruits and vegetables. This will ensure that you enjoy a greater diversity of beneficial plant chemicals while offering you eye-appealing meals.

**Benefits of Fruits and Vegetable**

There are many reasons why you need to add vegetables and fruits to your diet. Vegetables and fruits are critical to promoting good health and they need to be the foundation of a healthy diet. If you're not having sufficient amount of fruits and vegetables in your diet, then you need to increase your daily intake right now.

Vegetables and fruits are loaded with essential vitamins, fiber, disease-fighting phytochemicals, and minerals. This means that when you add plenty of vegetables and fruits to your diet, it can significantly lower your risk of high blood pressure, certain cancers, heart disease and type II diabetes. Phytochemicals are often related to color – vegetables and fruits which has different colors such as red, blue-purple, white, green, yellow-orange, all contain their combination of phytochemicals and nutrients which work together to keep you healthy.

Vegetables and fruits serve as one of the best ways to keep your body energized, especially when you consider the busy lives we live. Since some fruits don't require any form of cooking, they are easy to eat on-the-go which is perfect for our busy lives.

**Varieties of Fruit**

Fruits generally contain seed and they are the fleshy, sweet, and edible part of a plant. Most fruits are eaten raw while some can be cooked too. They come in several flavors, colors and shapes. Examples of some fruits that you can enjoy include:

- ✓ Tropical and exotic like mangoes and bananas
- ✓ Apples and pears
- ✓ Stone fruit - apricots, plums, nectarines, and peaches
- ✓ Tomatoes and avocados
- ✓ Citrus - grapefruits, limes, oranges, and mandarins
- ✓ Melons - rockmelons, honeydew melons, and watermelons
- ✓ Berries - Raspberries, passion fruit, strawberries, kiwifruit and blueberries

**Types of Healthy Vegetables**

Also, you will find vegetables in many varieties and they are generally grouped into families or biological groups such as:

- ✓ Edible plant stem - Celery and asparagus
- ✓ Leafy green - Spinach, silverbeet and lettuce
- ✓ Allium - Garlic, shallot and onion
- ✓ Cruciferous - cauliflower, broccoli, cabbage, Brussels sprouts
- ✓ Root - Sweet potato, potato and yam
- ✓ Marrow - Cucumber, zucchini, and pumpkin

**The Nutrients in Vegetables and Fruits**

The primary reason why it's important to add vegetables and fruits to your diet is that they provide nutrients that are crucial for the health and maintenance of your body. Let's take a look at the nutritional content of vegetables and fruits: vegetables are a vital source of many nutrients such as dietary fiber, vitamin A, vitamin C, folate (folic acid), and potassium.

The dietary fiber which you get from vegetables helps to reduce blood cholesterol levels and this, in turn, may lower risk of heart disease. Also, fiber is essential for good bowel function and it helps to reduce constipation and diverticulosis. When you eat fiber-containing foods such as fruits and vegetables, it provides you with a feeling of fullness with fewer calories.

Vegetables are generally low in fat and calories and they don't have cholesterol, but when you add sauces or seasoning, then they may indirectly add calories and cholesterol.

## Tips for Selecting and Eating more Vegetables and Fruits

What are some of the barriers to enjoying the power of produce? One of such barriers is the perception by most people that fruits and vegetables are expensive, but that's not necessarily so. When you buy most of these produce during their season, they are usually not expensive. Most importantly, when you consider the health implications of not eating fruits and vegetables, then you will discover that no price is too much to stay strong and healthy.

Other reasons why people don't eat much vegetables and fruits include the preparation time, old habits, and unfamiliarity. In order to maximize nutrients and appeal, you need to purchase and serve different varieties of fruits and vegetables. In fact, one of the best ways to increase your intake of fruits and vegetables is to buy the ones that are in season and also choose them based on their quality and freshness.

1.  **Eat them in seasons** - When you buy and eat fresh and high-quality fruits and vegetables, you are leveraging nature's provision for us to get a healthy mix of nutrients and plant chemicals.
2.  **Position your fruit where you can easily see it** - Strategically place various ready-to-eat washed whole fruits in a neat plate or you can also store chopped colorful fruits in a glass bowl in your refrigerator. This will easily tempt a sweet tooth.
3.  **Try to explore the produce aisle and go for something new** - The key to a healthy diet is variety and color. So, as much as possible, you need to get at least a serving from different categories such as yellow or orange fruits and vegetables, green leafy vegetables, legumes (beans), red fruits and peas.
4.  **Set a Goal** - If you have not made fruits and vegetables a major item in your menu, then you need to set that goal right now. Begin by eating just one extra vegetable and fruit per day and as soon as you're used to it, then add another one and keep increasing until you have achieved your goal.
5.  **Understand your needs** - You need to understand your vegetable and fruit needs first, but if this is difficult to do, just eat more. When it comes to fruits and vegetables, more is better!

6.  Fill half of your plate with vegetables and fruits at every meal and snack.

7.  **Substitute -** You can substitute vegetables and fruits in any meal since they contain lower calories than most foods.

8.  **Always stay stocked -** As much as possible, try to stock frozen and canned vegetables and fruits for quick meal preparation. When buying canned fruit and veggies, choose the ones without cream sauces, added sugar, syrup, as well as ingredients that may increase your calories intake.

9.  **Add More -** Cultivate the habit of adding extra fruits and vegetables to dishes even when they have already been added.

10. **Steam and flavor -** Add variety to your meals by eating steamed vegetables. You can add flavor with low-calorie or low-fat dressings as well as herbs and spices.

**Ideas for eating veggies and fruits**

**Breakfast**

✓ When taking cereal, add bananas, berries or raisins.

✓ Eat melon, grapefruit or other fruits.

✓ Take 6 oz. sglass of juice and ensure that the juice is 100 percent fruit or vegetable juice without excess sugar or sodium. Avoid "fruit drink," "punch," or "cocktail."

✓ Add chopped up veggies to your potatoes or eggs like green, onions, celery, or red bell peppers.

**Lunch**

✓ Add vegetables like sprouts, tomato, avocado, or cucumber to your sandwich.

✓ Eat a plate of vegetable soup. When buying it, check out the food labels and select the product that has the lowest level of sodium you can find. Preferably, you can also make soup from scratch. We shall look at the effects of excess salt and how to cut down on your salt and sugar intake in chapter five.

✓ Have a fruit or vegetable salad with lunch.

✓ Instead of chips, you can have a piece of fruit or raw veggie sticks.

**Snack Ideas**

✓ Add dried fruits such as dates, dried apricots, or raisins to your pocket or purse.

✓ During hot days, munch on a bowl of frozen fruits or vegetables like bananas, grapes or peas.

✓ Ensure you have raw veggie sticks close to you like red bell peppers, carrots, green beans or celery.

✓ Eat any kind of fresh fruit such as banana, kiwi, grapes, apple, orange, etc.

**Dinner Ideas**

✓ Add chopped vegetable such as garlic, celery, and onions when cooking beans, stew, soup, spaghetti sauce, and rice.

✓ Add a side of microwaved or steamed vegetable.

✓ While cooking rice, you can add some frozen peas during the last three minutes of cooking.

# Chapter Three

# Choosing the Best Kind of Food - Organic, Natural & GMO Foods

It's not really enough for you to understand the importance of nutrition in the foods you eat; you also need to know the quality of the ingredients you use. The common rule for everyone when shopping is; if you're unable to pronounce the names on the label, then it's probably not good for you. You must understand that processed food poses long and short term risks to your body.

Unfortunately, most labels fail to disclose the real ingredients and items used in the preparation of foods. So, any generic or vague term like "natural flavor" is often an indication of a preservative or chemical. It's usually difficult to determine the quantity of sugar and fats in processed foods. Whether you see artificial flavors or natural flavors on the label, they all contain the same chemicals but were manufactured/produced differently.

The reason why processed foods are not good for your health is that they are stripped of their nutrients and this ends up eliminating their natural flavor and that's why the manufacturers need to add artificial or "natural" flavors to the foods. You should understand that these flavors are not actually derived from the food product, rather they are often derived from animal byproducts and in some cases, chemicals.

Also, unless otherwise stated, when you find the word dextrose or soy in your nutritional label, then, you know that it's GMO. You must have come across some signs while shopping like organic, natural and GMO-free foods. That's actually the focus of this chapter – how healthy are GMO foods? There is a significant difference between the three labels earlier mentioned. If you truly want to prioritize the quality of the food you eat, then you need to understand what GMO, organic, and natural foods mean.

## Organic

Generally, this has to do with how agricultural products are grown and processed. This regulation varies from country to country; for instance, in the United States, all organic crops have to be grown without bioengineered genes (GMO), sewage sludge-based fertilizers, synthetic pesticides and petroleum-based fertilizers. You can find out what's obtained in your country. Also, when it comes to livestock that was raised for dairy products, eggs and meat, they must have access to the outdoors and fed with organic food. Such animals may not be given any animal by-products, growth hormones or antibiotics.

### *So, what are some of the benefits of organic foods?*

Understand that the way your food is grown or raised can significantly affect your mental and emotional health. In fact, it also has an impact on your environment. Generally, organic foods usually possess more beneficial nutrients like antioxidants than those that were conventionally grown.

Most people with allergies to chemicals, preservatives and foods usually find their symptoms either lessen or are totally eliminated when they begin to eat just organic foods. So, when you choose organic foods, you stand to enjoy some of these benefits:

✓ **Organic foods are usually fresher -** The reason why organic foods are fresher is that they don't contain preservatives that are meant to make them last much longer. Most times, organic foods are (though not in all cases) produced on smaller farms close to the shop where they are sold.

✓ **Animals that are organically grown are not given growth hormones** - When livestock are fed animal byproducts, it significantly increases the risk of mad cow disease (BSE). In addition, the use of antibiotics for animals can lead to the creation of antibiotic-resistant strains of bacteria. Animals that are raised organically are often given more space to move around and they have access to outdoors, which ensures that they are healthy.

✓ **Organic produce also contains less pesticides** - In conventional agriculture, chemicals like herbicides, insecticides, and fungicides are used in growing the food we eat. Unfortunately, residues remain on (and in) the food we eat which is harmful to the body. Organic foods contain far less resides of such chemicals than the others.

✓ **Organic farming helps our environment** - With the gradual increase in global warming, organic farming practice helps to reduce soil erosion, conserve water, reduce pollution, use less energy, and increase soil fertility. Also, farming without pesticides favors nearby birds and animals and people living close to farms.

✓ **Organic meat and dairy contain certain nutrients** - According to a result of a 2016 European study, there is a significant increase (as high as 50 percent) in the levels of some nutrients such as omega-3 fatty acids in organic meat and milk compared to their conventionally raised counterparts.

**Locally Grown Foods**

Okay, things are getting more interesting right now. Unlike the organic standards, local foods don't have a specific definition. So, such foods could be grown in your state, local community, region, or country. You often find foods that were grown close to home in places like a farmer's market and they also have several advantages. One of the benefits of locally grown food is that the money derived from the sales stays within the local economy.

Instead of releasing more money to marketing and distribution, more money goes directly to the farmer. Locally grown foods are often fresher and full of flavor since they are harvested when ripe.

**GMOs**

There has always been a strong and controversial debate regarding the effects of GMOs on health as well as our environment. The main reason for GMOs is that they are engineered to ensure that crops are resistant to herbicides or produce insecticide. In fact, much of the sweet corn that's presently being consumed in the US, for instance, are genetically engineered to make them resistant to the herbicide Roundup and also to produce its insecticide, Bt Toxin.

Also, in the US, some of the crops you will find GMOs include soybeans, squash, papaya, canola, alfalfa and zucchini. They are present in many breakfast cereals and the majority of the processed foods we eat. When you see corn syrup or soy lecithin as part of the ingredients on a package, then it's most likely that they contain GMOs.

Since the introduction of GMOs, there has also been a significant increase (about 15 times) in the use of toxic herbicides such as Roundup (glyphosate). Although the World Health Organization announced that glyphosate is "probably carcinogenic to humans," a lot of controversy regarding the extent of health risk posed by the use of pesticides still exists. So, the question that comes to mind here is, are GMOs really safe?

Although biotech companies that engineer GMOs, as well as the US Food and Drug Administration (FDA), insist that they are safe, a good number of safety advocates have expressed their concerns regarding GMOs. They are of the view that no long term studies have ever been carried out to confirm how safe it is to use GMOs.

In addition, several animal studies have given some indications that consuming GMOs may lead to slowed brain growth, thickening of the digestive tract and may also cause internal organ damage. GMOs have also been linked to gastrointestinal problems in humans and increased food allergies for some people. Although some people believe that altering the DNA of an animal or plant can increase the risk of cancer, research to prove this has so far been inconclusive.

**Are Organic Foods Pesticide Free?**

As earlier mentioned, organic foods have lower levels of pesticides, which means that they are not also completely free from pesticides. Organic farms still make use of pesticides, but the types they use are the naturally-derived pesticides. Most conventional commercial farms make use of synthetic pesticides and natural pesticides are believed to be less toxic, though some of them have proven to have health risks as well. But when you eat organic foods, you significantly reduce your exposure to harmful pesticides.

**Vegetables and Fruits where the Organic label Matters Most**

According to the results of an analysis of government pesticide testing in the US, the Environmental Working Group which is a nonprofit organization has released the list of fruits and vegetables which have the highest levels of pesticides. This also means that these are produce you might consider buying organic:

- ✓ Grapes
- ✓ Peaches
- ✓ Summer squash
- ✓ Strawberries
- ✓ Cucumbers
- ✓ Cherry tomatoes
- ✓ Apples
- ✓ Sweet bell peppers
- ✓ Imported nectarines
- ✓ Hot peppers
- ✓ Kale/collard greens
- ✓ Spinach

**Vegetables and Fruits you don't have to Buy Organic**

Also, regarded as the "clean 15," some of the conventionally-grown vegetables and fruits that are low in pesticides include:

- ✓ Papaya
- ✓ Grapefruit
- ✓ Onion
- ✓ Sweet potatoes
- ✓ Asparagus
- ✓ Cabbage
- ✓ Pineapple
- ✓ Eggplant
- ✓ Mushrooms
- ✓ Sweet peas (frozen)
- ✓ Cantaloupe

✓ Kiwi

✓ Sweet corn

✓ Mango

Apart from fruits and vegetables, you can also buy organic eggs, dairy and meat provided you can afford them. Although some major health organizations are of the view that eating saturated fat from any source increases the risk of heart disease, some nutrition experts believe that eating organic dairy products and organic grass-fed meat doesn't have the same risks. They believe that the problem isn't the saturated fats, but the unnatural diet of animals that are industrially-raised which includes hormones, medication and corn.

I believe you're already interested in buying more organic foods. But don't forget that they are not cheap. So, how do you ensure that you enjoy foods that are natural and healthy without spending much?

✓ **Try to shop at farmers' market -** Regardless of your location, you will certainly find several cities and small towns which have a weekly farmer's market. This is where local farmers sell their produce at a discount to grocery stores and such markets are open-air street markets. You can buy fresh farm produce at fair rates when you visit such markets.

✓ **Always try to buy in season -** Obviously, vegetables and fruits are usually cheapest and freshest during their season. So, if you want to buy the freshest food possible, try to find out when produce is being delivered to your market.

Always bear in mind that organic doesn't necessarily equal healthy. For instance, one marketing strategy you will find in the food industry is making junk food to sound healthy. However, organic baked goods, snacks and desserts often contain high levels of fat, calories, salt and sugar. You still need to at least read the food labels carefully to know what each food contains before buying them.

Choosing organic isn't just the best way to eat a healthy and nutritious diet; it also ensures that we promote a healthy environment. If you genuinely want to encourage a sustainable future for our children and grandchildren, then you need to shop organic. You will be sure that you're not buying pretty-looking junk-filled foods that are less nutritious. Organic practices support both farming and harvesting processes that ensure healthy and fertile soil. Clean, organic practices ensure that animal and vegetative life remain intact; it's also in harmony with our natural environment and helps to maintain a peaceful and symbiotic relationship.

# Chapter Four
# Switching to a Healthy Diet

Living a healthy lifestyle is crucial to having a quality life. Most people understand that they need to make changes to their diet, but are often scared of making the right changes. Switching to a healthy diet shouldn't be an all or nothing proposition as some health experts say. In fact, there is no need for you to be perfect and you shouldn't completely eliminate the foods you enjoy. That's why I added the Harvard eating Pyramid earlier to help you understand the kinds of food you should eat in moderation and the ones you're free to eat as much as you can.

Besides, you don't even need to make the changes also at once because it often leads to cheating or entirely abandoning your new eating plan. In line with the approach of this book, you can make a few changes at a time. Remember, you can achieve more in the long term without feeling being overwhelmed by a major change in diet or feeling deprived. You can approach it as taking several small and manageable steps and as you continue to make the changes, they will become habits. Once you have created a habit, then you can add more healthy choices too.

## So how do you set yourself up for Success?

Eating a healthier diet doesn't necessarily have to be a complicated affair; try to keep things as simple as possible. For instance, rather than focusing mainly on counting your calories intake, you can consider your diet in terms of freshness, variety and color. Also, focus on avoiding certain foods like packaged and processed foods, then focus more on fresh ingredients as often as possible. Consider the tips below when setting yourself up for success.

## #1. Make the right changes

The process of switching from unhealthy foods in your diet to healthy ones requires that you replace unhealthy foods with healthy alternatives. For instance, switching from fried chicken to grilled salmon (replacing trans-fat with healthy fats) will positively make a difference in your health. But deciding to switch animal fats for refined carbohydrates like eating a donut instead of bacon, won't reduce your risk for heart disease and won't even increase your mood. So, make the right changes.

## #2. Endeavor to prepare your meals

You can easily take charge of the kind of foods you're eating and monitor the ingredients that go into the preparation of your food by cooking more of your meals at home. This will also make you eat fewer calories, avoid unhealthy fats of packaged and takeout foods, chemicals in additives and added sugar. These are some of the things that make you feel tired, irritable, bloated and can further worsen the symptoms of stress, anxiety and depression.

## #3. Always Read Labels

Most times, all we just do when shopping is to look at the brand name. We don't take time to check out what is in our food, and the manufacturers often hide large amounts of unhealthy fats or sugar in packaged foods which they claim to be healthy. When shopping, carefully read the labels on the food and as earlier mentioned, if you're unable to pronounce the names you see on the food, then it's probably not healthy enough for you.

## #4. Observe how you feel after eating

When you observe how you feel after eating, you will foster healthy habits and tastes. Interestingly, the healthier the food you eat, the better you will feel after eating a meal. On the other hand, you are likely going to feel nauseous, uncomfortable or even drained of energy when you consume more junk foods.

## #5. Embracing Moderation

Most times, we get tempted to eat more food than we really need, especially when the meal is tasty. But when you practice moderation, then you just need to eat as much food as required by your body. At the end of a meal, you should feel satisfied and not stuffed. So, moderation for most of us has to do with eating less food than we currently do; however, moderation doesn't imply that you should eliminate the foods you love. For instance, you can consider eating bacon for breakfast once every week as moderation if followed by a healthy lunch and dinner instead of a sausage pizza or a box of donuts.

## #6. Focus more on Smaller Portions

Recently, serving sizes have increased significantly. Rather than choose an entree, go for a starter when dining out; you can even split a dish with a friend and avoid ordering anything supersized. One of the ways to control your portion sizes is to use visual cues. For example, you can make your serving of fish, meat or chicken to be the size of a deck of cards and half a cup of rice, pasta, mashed potato, is approximately the size of a traditional bulb.

You can also trick your brain into thinking that your food is a larger portion by serving your meals on smaller plates. You can add more leafy greens or some fruits if you don't feel satisfied after eating your meal.

Sometimes, your focus should be not on what you eat but how much of the food you're eating. For instance, it's generally believed that avocados are very healthy and they have so many health benefits in terms of healthy fats and nutrients. Well, on the flip side, avocados are dense in calories and this implies that eating three avocados each day may not be a healthy habit. So, take note of the following tips to help with portion control:

✓ Listen to your hunger cue
✓ Avoid eating whenever you feel stressed
✓ Take plenty of water and other healthy fluids
✓ Make use of portion-control containers to store your meals
✓ Maintain a food journal or diary
✓ Use portion-control plates anytime you're eating at home
✓ Prepare and eat healthy smoothies
✓ Plan your meals every week
✓ As much as possible, limit distractions during meal times
✓ Avoid fun-sized candy bars as well as other treats
✓ Chew your food at least five times before you swallow them
✓ Drink water even before you get thirsty

## #7. Reduce Snack foods at home

Take note of the kind of foods you keep at hand because you will find it more difficult to eat in moderation if there are unhealthy snacks and treats close to you. Rather than have unhealthy snacks close to you, opt for healthy choices and any time you want to reward yourself, then go out and get them.

## #8. Avoid Thinking of certain foods as "off-limits"

The moment you completely ban certain foods, you will naturally desire such foods and feel like you've failed once you give in to temptation. So, instead of banning unhealthy foods, start by reducing portion sizes of such foods and don't eat them as often as you did before. As you gradually begin to reduce your intake of unhealthy foods, you may also begin to notice that you now think less of them and only indulge in them occasionally.

## #9. Control emotional eating

Most times, the reason why we eat is not really to satisfy hunger; instead, most of us eat food just to relieve stress or even cope with unpleasant emotions such as boredom, loneliness and sadness. When you learn healthier ways to manage stress and emotions, you will be able to regain control over your feelings and the food you eat.

# Chapter Five
# Be Mindful of Your Salt & Sugar Intake

When you pick up any kind of food in the grocery store, you're likely going to find some amounts of sodium and sugar. Although you may not be on any restrictive diet, in line with the goal of this book, you need to know how much salt or sugar you may be consuming unknowingly. But why do you need to pay attention to the quantity of salt and sugar you consume?

**Is Too Much Salt Dangerous?**

Experts are of the view that we actually need salt in our body, but we also need to watch our salt intake. Averagely, it's estimated that people consume between 9,000-12,000 milligrams of sodium daily. Interestingly, this is three times the recommended amount. The maximum recommended amount of sodium per day is 2,300 milligrams and the most preferred is 1,500 milligrams, especially for adults with high blood pressure.

Although there are no side effects of eating too much salt for most people, it doesn't eliminate the fact that salt intake has some negative effects on the body, especially when taken above the recommended amount. Some of the health effects of eating excess salt include:

✓ **Heart health:** For people with heart disease or congestive heart failure, the consumption of excess salt can lead to fluid retention and this will, in turn, result in shortness of breath.

✓ **Blood pressure:** The excess intake of sodium is also linked to high blood pressure or hypertension. In fact, lowering salt intake to 5,000-6,000 milligrams per day has proven to lower blood pressure.

✓ **Diabetes:** Although eating too much salt is not directly connected to blood sugar, it actually increases the risk of complication from diabetes.

✓ **Kidney function:** For people with kidney disease, adding too much salt to your diet may also cause you to retain fluid and this will lead to weight gain and bloating.

You may not really be adding much salt to your food when preparing them at home, but that doesn't mean you're not exceeding your daily salt limit. Approximately 90 percent of the salt we consume comes from sodium chloride which we commonly call table salt. But a large portion of the salt most people consume are in manufactured foods and not the ones people sprinkle out of salt shakers.

Did you know that a single serving of potato chips contains several hundred mg of sodium while a serving of salad dressing can have as much as those chips? You need to understand that the main cause of salt in your diet is the dietary sodium which comes with most processed foods.

### *So, how can you reduce your salt intake?*

One of the easiest ways to reduce the amount of salt in your diet is to avoid adding salt to your already cooked meal and also avoid processed foods. When buying foods, it's crucial to take a closer look at the nutritional labels. Avoid foods that have high salt content such as pickles and bacon. By reducing your intake of salt and embracing low-sodium foods, you can significantly lower blood pressure. But, this isn't an easy task because foods with close to zero salt tend to be tasteless.

However, the good news here is that once you're able to control your salt intake, your body will also become more sensitive to the salt in most foods. This implies that you will no longer be comfortable eating most processed foods since they will become too salty for your taste. Don't forget that it's possible for you to enjoy lower sodium foods without even missing the flavor. The easiest way to reduce your salt intake is to eat unprocessed food which has little or no added salt. You can enjoy low-salt recipes at home by experimenting with various spices in your cupboard instead of using your salt shaker.

You can also consider some of these useful tips to help you reduce your salt intake:

- ✓ You can buy tuna and pulses tinned in water instead of brine and in case food is tinned in brine, rinse it properly before using it to eliminate as much salt as possible.
- ✓ As much as possible, don't add salt when cooking and if you do, then ensure that it's added at the end of the cooking time. Then gradually reduce the amount you add and over time, your taste buds will quickly adjust.
- ✓ When buying food, go for reduced salt options as earlier mentioned.
- ✓ If you're going to use canned vegetables like sweetcorn, choose the ones that are canned in water with no added sugar and salt.
- ✓ Instead of using salt, you can also experiment with spices, and herbs to add flavor to your cooking.

## Moderate Intake of Sugar

Naturally, sugar can be found in some foods like vegetables and fruits and it can also be added during the preparation of food. Generally, we can find sugar in almost everything that's not real food. You are not likely going to find sugar in vegetable-based proteins such as nuts and seeds. Also, other foods such as animal-based proteins like chicken, beef, fish or pork don't have sugars.

Foods that contain natural sugar include fruits and vegetables and a significant portion of the sugar and sweeteners we consume are found in convenience foods and soft drinks. Most of us consume more than the recommended amount of sugar and most sugary foods are usually high in calories, which results in weight gain and tooth decay. It's most likely that you're already aware that eating too much sugar is harmful, but you have not been able to stop excess sugar intake.

In the US, for instance, the average American consume an average of 20 teaspoons of added sugars each day against the six teaspoons that was recommended for women and 9 for men. This excludes the sugar consumed from natural foods such as vegetables, milk and fruits. The main sources of added sugar include baked foods, sweetened dairy, candy and sugary drinks. But there are also other sources that we may not even notice such as bread, protein bars, and tomato sauce and they often make it easy for us to consume surplus sugar.

What further complicates this is the fact that most added sugars just like salt are difficult to identify on nutrition labels. The reason is that they are often listed under different names like agave nectar, sucrose, cane juice, corn syrup, palm sugar, etc. Regardless of the name it's called, one thing remains true — sugar is sugar and it can affect your body negatively in various ways. Some of the health challenges of consuming excess sugar include:

✓ **Influences your brain:** When you consume sugar, it gives your brain a significant surge of a feel-good chemical known as dopamine and this is why you have a higher tendency to desire a candy bar at 3 pm instead of an apple or carrot. Since your brain doesn't get such effect from whole foods like fruits and vegetables, your brain will begin to crave more and more sugar just to experience the same pleasurable feeling.

✓ **It can worsen joint pain:** Consuming lots of sugar has shown to worsen joint pain as a result of the inflammation they cause in the body. Also, several studies have revealed that the intake of sugar can increase your risk of developing rheumatoid arthritis.

✓ **Affects your sexual health:** Among the most common side effects of chronically high levels of sugar in our bloodstream is that it's capable of making men impotent. The reason is that it affects your circulatory system and this is what controls blood flow all through the body and it has to work properly before you can get an erection.

✓ **Excess Sugar can increase your Body Weight:** I guess this isn't news to you anymore. The excess intake of sugar can increase your weight. According to research, individuals who consume sugar-sweetened beverages seem to gain more weight and are at a higher risk for type II diabetes than people who don't.

✓ **May increase the risk of heart disease:** Diets that contain a high amount of sugar have been linked with an increased risk of several diseases such as heart disease which is the number one cause of death around the world. According to research, high-sugar diets can cause obesity, high triglyceride, inflammation, blood sugar, and high blood pressure levels. All these are risk factors for heart disease.

### *So, how can you reduce your sugar intake?*

To help reduce your level of sugar intake, take note of the tips below:

✓ Always buy reduced-sugar versions of foods like sauces, yogurt, sweetcorn, cereal and baked beans.

✓ For a healthy dessert, drizzle fruit purees on top of fat-free Greek yogurt. You can also make fruit purees using naturally sweet fruits like mango.

✓ Instead of using sugar, make use of dried or chopped fruit to sweeten desserts.

✓ Make use of spices as well as other flavors instead of adding sugar. You can bring out fruit flavors by using lemon or orange zest while nutmeg or vanilla are great for adding sweetness.

✓ Instead of sugary drinks, drink water. You can reduce the level of calories you consume by drinking water or other unsweetened beverages. Drinks like sports drinks, soda, energy drinks, etc., are the main sources of added sugar and calories. To get some flavor, you can add lime, a slice of lemon, or watermelon to your glass of water.

The introduction of various kinds of junk foods has actually conditioned most of us to crave sugar and salt. However, our tongue is capable of tasting various flavors other than salt and sugar. You can successfully shift your food habits from eating excess salt and sugar by gradually mixing up with other types of flavors. This will significantly reduce your taste bud's dependence on salt or sugar.

# Chapter Six
# Health Benefits of Slow-Eating

Did you know that when you eat slowly, your food will digest better? There are several benefits of slow-eating and we shall be looking at how it will enhance your health. When you eat slowly, you tend to feel more satisfied with every meal. On the other hand, your digestion will suffer when you rush your meals and your meals will be stressful. It sometimes appear as if each meal finished too soon and this may cause you to eat more and consuming large quantities of food even before your natural satiety signals appear.

At this point, you end up uncomfortable and overstuffed. So, why do you need to slow down your eating? Consider the busy world we live in; we're distracted, rushed, and too busy. Most of us really eat fast and rarely have sufficient time to savor our food and in some cases, chew the food properly. Take a look at some of the reasons why you need to eat slowly.

**1.  It enables you to sense satisfaction**

This is perhaps the greatest benefit of eating slowly; it gives your body sufficient time to recognize that you're full. Interestingly, it takes approximately 20 minutes from the beginning of a meal for your brain to send out signals of satiety to the rest parts of your body. Unfortunately, most people's meal don't even last as much as 20 minutes. Well, can you imagine the extra calories you could be taking in just because you failed to give your body enough time to inform you that you no longer need food?

Another aspect of sensing satisfaction is that eating slowly enables us to feel more satisfied and this is quite different from being "full." By slowing down when eating, you can savor a meal, observe the textures, tastes and appreciate every mindful bite. After such meals, you will leave the table feeling satisfied instead of feeling that you've fulfilled your obligation to your body.

## 2.  It Improves digestion

One way to understand digestion is to see it as a chain reaction. Once we see, smell or even think of food, we immediately begin to salivate in preparation to put the food in our mouth. The saliva in our mouth contains enzymes which helps to break down the food while moistening the mouth for easier swallowing. This will be followed by the remaining steps of the digestion process. So, whenever we rush this eating process, we usually compel our GI tract to handle food substances before it's fully ready.

Although surprises are awesome on our birthdays, they are not really great during digestion. In fact, researchers at the University of Rhode Island examined the effect of eating speed on the early stages of digestive processing. During the study, they observed 60 young adults as they ate their food:

✓ Fast eaters consumed 3.1 ounces per minute, took larger bites and didn't chew much before swallowing.
✓ Medium-speed eaters consumed 2.5 ounces of food every minute.
✓ Slow eaters consumed 2 ounces of food per minute.

A look at these finding revealed that not only are fast eater consuming more food at any given time, but the food they consume is also not properly processed. So, the foods that fast eaters consume simply land in their stomach in big lumps. Since digestion begins in the mouth, it will always be more difficult for your stomach to turn inadequately chewed food into chyme. Chyme is the liquid mix of hydrochloric acid, partially digested food, digestive enzymes and water which passes through the pyloric valve while it's about to be eliminated. One of the things that often leads to indigestion as well as other potential GI problems is food that isn't properly broken down into chyme.

## 3.   You Eat smaller portions without even trying

Generally, the majority of research on slow eating indicate that it helps us to eat less. So, this means that if you're trying to lose weight, then this is something you need to take seriously. According to another study at the University of Rhode Island, 30 normal-weight women were served lunch on two separate occasions. Both meals consist of an enormous plate of pasta, some Parmesan cheese, a tomato vegetable sauce as well as a glass of water.

The researchers asked the women to eat until the point of comfortable fullness. Also, during one of the visits, the researchers instructed the women to eat as quickly as possible and on other visits, participants were told to eat their food slowly and drop their utensils between bites. After comparing the difference in food consumption between the slowly eaten lunch and the quickly eaten lunch, they discovered that:

- ✓ The women consumed 646 calories in 9 minutes while eating quickly.
- ✓ When the participants ate slowly, they consumed 579 calories in 29 minutes.

This translates to a total of 67 calories less in extra 20 minutes. Well, what will this look like when you consider three meals per day? I guess you now see how the extra calories often add up. But that's not all, another interesting observation which the researchers made was that when the women ate their lunch quickly, they reported being hungrier an hour later than they did after eating their lunch slowly. This implies that not only did eating quickly lead to consuming more food; it also satisfied the women less. On the other hand, slow eating results in eating less food but offers us long-lasting satisfaction.

While learning to eat the right diets with the right nutrition, most of us tend to overlook the way we eat food. Considering our hectic and fast-paced lives, it's usually justifiable for us to rush our meals. However, it's one eating habit that we must replace with slow-eating because it doesn't favor us. It causes us to eat more food than we need and this results in lower satisfaction from eating, weight gain and poor digestion. When we replace our habit of rushing our food with slow-paced eating, it leads to better digestion, greater satisfaction after our meals and easier weight maintenance. Below are some tips to help you eat slowly.

- ✓ Choose more of high-fiber foods like fresh fruits and vegetables because you need to spend more time chewing them.
- ✓ When eating, sit down in a calm environment and avoid distractions. Avoid eating while watching TV, texting, or driving because you may not know when you exceed your body needs. So, focus on your food while eating.
- ✓ Drop your utensils between meals, then take a moment to breathe. You can even enjoy making nice conversation for a few minutes when eating with other people.
- ✓ Make use of smaller plates or different utensils like chopsticks.
- ✓ Look for someone else who is a slow eater and pace yourself to them. An ideal person could be the picky little kid or a chatty dinner companion who doesn't want to stop talking before taking a bite.
- ✓ Endeavor to set a minimum number of chews per bite. Although this will appear to be strange initially, you will be amazed at what you will discover when you try it.

✓ Create a timeframe to eat. Set aside at least 20-30 minutes for each meal – preferably longer at dinner. Avoid eating food as an inconvenience or whenever you get around to it. Remember, what you're doing when eating is that you're fueling your body and also spending good time with family and friends. So, it's an action that deserves an appointment.

When you discover that you're rushing, that's quite okay. But you need to change the habit, so drop your utensils and spend a minute bringing your attention to what you are doing. This process will require lots of practice if slow eating isn't habitual for you.

# Chapter Seven

# Water - An Essential Aspect of Your Diet

**Why You Need to Drink Water**

Obviously, every one of us needs water to survive, but how exactly does water intake help us? Well, as earlier mentioned, our body weight is approximately 60 percent water. Generally, our body makes use of water in all its organs, tissues and cells to help regulate its temperature while maintaining other bodily functions.

During the day, your body loses water via sweating, digestion and breathing and this explains why it's crucial to rehydrate by taking water and foods that also contain water. Several factors determine the amount of water you need and this includes your level of physical activity, the climate you live in and whether you have any health problems. Take a look at other functions of water in the body below:

**Water Helps Your Body to Eliminate Waste**

When you take adequate water, it helps your body to excrete waste through urination, defecation and perspiration. Water is used by the kidneys and liver to flush out waste just like your intestines. Also, water can prevent you from being constipated by softening your stools and moving the food you ate through your intestinal tract. But always bear in mind that there isn't any evidence to prove that increased fluid intake can cure constipation.

**Helps to keep you Hydrated**

As earlier mentioned, you lose water during the day, especially when you engage in vigorous exercise and sweat profusely during high heat. Also, when you have a fever or an illness which causes diarrhea or vomiting, it can cause you to lose fluids too. Regardless of the reason why you're losing fluids, as long as you're losing fluids, it's crucial that you also increase the intake of fluids to help your body restore its natural hydration levels.

Also, your doctor may suggest that you take more fluids to help resolve certain health conditions such as urinary tract stones or bladder infections. You may have to consult your doctor regarding your fluid intake if you are pregnant or nursing because your body will be using more fluids than normal.

**Water Helps to Protect Your Spinal Cord, Tissues and Joints**

Apart from helping to quench our thirst and regulate the temperature of our body, it also helps to keep the tissues in your body moist. We don't always feel comfortable when our mouth, eyes and nose gets dry. You can retain optimum levels of moisture in the sensitive parts of your body and bones, the brain and the blood by keeping your body hydrated. Actually, water helps to act as a lubricant; it helps to protect the spinal cord and acts as a cushion for the joints.

**Water is Essential for Digestion**

The digestion of the food we eat starts with saliva in our mouth, which is composed of water. Digestion relies greatly on enzymes which can be found in saliva and they help to break down liquid and food and also dissolve minerals as well as other nutrients. When there is proper digestion, then nutrients and minerals become more accessible to our body. Also, water is crucial in the digestion of soluble fiber, which positively improves the health of our bowel by making well-formed and soft stools that we can easily pass.

**It Boosts Energy**

The intake of water may also activate your metabolism; in fact, a boost in metabolism has actually been associated with a positive impact on your energy level. According to a study, drinking 500 milliliters of water boosted the metabolic rate by 30 percent both in men and women, and these effects seem to last over one hour.

*So, how much water should you take?*

There isn't a specific quantity when it comes to the quantity of water you should drink daily. Well, it's been discovered that many individuals meet their daily hydration needs by taking water whenever they are thirsty. But when you're unsure of your level of hydration, take a look at your urine. A clear urine is an indication that you're well-hydrated while a dark one simply means that you're likely dehydrated.

## Common Signs of Hydration

First, you should understand that the regulation of the input and output of water is one of the key ways of maintaining proper hydration. Water is required by our body for basic metabolism, osmoregulation and organ function. The moment there is a greater water output compared to water intake, then blood pressure will drop. This will lead to a physiological chain reaction that will trigger thirst and further reduce the production of urine.

Generally, men need a daily intake of 13 cups of fluid to enable them to stay hydrated. On the other hand, women need about nine cups each day also to maintain hydration. Some of the fluid intake includes milk, juices, water, coffee and other beverages. One primary indicator of a body that's properly hydrated is a clear urine that's light in color. Interestingly, adequate hydration results in less than one percent weight loss from pre-workout weight and a weight loss, which is over one percent may likely be an indication of dehydration.

Those who are very active tend to sweat more and they actually place more demand on their muscles than those who are less active. Also, such people would require more than the average recommended water level to stay hydrated.

**Common Indicators of Dehydration**

The primary sign of insufficient hydration is thirst; however, there are other symptoms of dehydration such as dizziness, urine that's darker than normal, fatigue, confusion, and lethargy. For older adults, dehydration can lead to severe health issues because the sensation of thirst tends to diminish as we grow older. According to ACSM Health and Fitness Journal, a one to two percent loss of water can cause mild dehydration, which has negative effects on critical thinking, on our mood, reaction time and short-term memory.

## How to Stay Hydrated

To avoid dehydration, you need to make hydration a healthy habit. Some of the tips that can help you achieve this include:

- ✓ **Add some color:** If you find plain water not to be palatable, then you can make use of other colorful ideas to make it more appealing. For instance, you can add slices of lime or lemon, cucumber or orange slices, berries or a few springs of mint or basil to your water to give it some color and flavor.
- ✓ **Begin and end your day with water:** Just before you grab a cup of coffee, first drink a glass of water and while reading a book or engaging

in other bedtime rituals, sip on water as well. Have a glass of water at your nightstand so you won't find it hard to drink once you're getting set to sleep. Note that drinking much water at night may affect the quality of your sleep, which may lead to weight gain.

✓ **Make drinking water convenient:** Place a refillable bottle of water at your desk, in your car, kitchen sink, bag, or other places where you visit daily. You are likely to drink more water when you have it close at hand.

✓ **Add water-rich foods in your diet:** Some foods like broth-based soups, oatmeal, fruits, vegetables, and beans have high water content. When you add them to your diet, they can also help to keep your body hydrated and even give you a feeling of fullness.

✓ **Always drink a glass of water after your meal or a snack:** Considering the busy and stressful times we live in right now, it's often easy to forget to drink water. One way to overcome this problem and stay hydrated throughout the day is to ensure that you drink water after eating.

# Chapter Eight
# Sleep Is As Crucial as Exercise & Diet

Many people fail to understand that sleep is actually on the same level of importance as exercise and diet. Although we have been focusing on the importance of nutrition, a healthy diet without adequate rest is incomplete. Most people often make efforts to ensure that they have an awesome nutritional plan, supplementation regimen, and a well-structured exercise program. Unfortunately, less focus is placed on sleep as well as the quality of sleep.

Even if you fail to eat properly, you can still expect to live up to 75 years, but if you fail to sleep, you're likely going to die within a couple of weeks. So, sleep is quite essential to health and survival. Did you know that the Guinness World Record for sleep deprivation is 11 days? Most of us wouldn't even dare to break that record soon even though parents of newborns and medical students feel that they might be inadvertently trying.

What you need to ask yourself right now is: are you sleeping optimally? What are the implications of poor sleep quality to your body's composition as well as your eating habits? Are you failing to make nutritious food choices because of late nights in front of the computer, smartphone or TV?

## Facts about Sleep

Generally, the average adult sleeps for about seven hours each night and 33 percent of people get fewer than 6.5 hours of sleep per night. I guess this explains why the world appears to be cranky and often distracted. It's been discovered that women sleep a bit more than men and individuals that have a high level of body fat tend to sleep less than others with normal body fat.

Did you also know that studies have confirmed that individuals who sleep for less than six hours each night gain almost twice as much weight within six years as others who sleep for 7-8 hours each night? Well, if you think you can reduce your weight by sleeping excessively, then you're wrong as well because it isn't necessarily better. Studies have shown that people who sleep for over 9 hours each night have similar body composition outcomes as those with less than six hours.

**Sleep and our Body Composition**

In the United States, for instance, a 2005 study suggested that the obesity epidemic may be partly caused by a corresponding decrease in the average number of sleep hours. The study discovered that staying awake beyond midnight tend to increase the possibility of someone having obesity and people between the ages of 32 and 49 who had less than seven hours of sleep per night are more likely to be obese.

Another study which followed the growth of over 9,000 children from birth discovered that those who slept the least when they were 30 months old were significantly more likely to be obese when they reached seven than the children who had more sleeping time. There are many possible reasons why the lack of sleep could influence body fat. For instance, it could be as a result of a decreased thyroid-stimulating hormone (TSH), growth hormone (GH), and increased cortisol, especially in the evening.

Also, chronic sleep restriction leads to elevated sympathetic nerve activity as well as a slow insulin response. This actually is the storm of peripheral effects to foster obesity:

- ✓  Lowered leptin
- ✓  Lowered glucose tolerance (GT)
- ✓  Increased sympathovagal balance
- ✓  Insufficient thyroid-stimulating hormone (TSH)
- ✓  Increased evening and nocturnal cortisol levels

On the other hand, the lack of sleep may also cause you to have more body fat just because when you spend more time staying awake, you end up eating more. You begin to appreciate those junk food commercials more at 1 am when you're supposed to be asleep. Also, scientists have speculated that deregulation of appetite hormones could also be one good reason why sleep deprivation may lead to weight gains.

Apart from the impact of sleep on weight, having less than 7.5 hours of sleep potentially exposes you to a greater risk of sudden cardiac death, stroke and heart attack. In addition, with the increase in your weight due to insufficient sleep, you're exposed to issues like insulin resistance (IR) glucose intolerance and type II diabetes.

## Tips for Improving your Sleep Quality & Quantity

Since most results from various research findings indicate that sleep duration is closely linked with obesity, you need to find a suitable sleeping strategy and make it a part of your healthy living as well as good nutrition routine. Our world is a busy one, and you'll always have more opportunities to do things than to sleep – extended work shifts, the internet, social media, 24-hour cable/satellite TV, 24-hour shopping, family commitments and several others.

However, don't forget that we also have the option most of the time to choose what we do. This implies that the lack of sleep often reflects our priorities instead of real constraints. So, if you're genuinely concerned about the quality of your sleep, then you need to start accessing the quality of your sleep right now – where do you stand?

Just as it's crucial to have a food journal or diary, it's been recommended by sleep experts that we have a sleep diary. Monitor your sleep to find out whether you are getting up to 7-9 hours of sleep each night. If you're not getting sufficient sleep, then what are the causes? Medication, poor sleep hygiene, or other negative habits? Discover the main reasons why you're not having enough sleep at night.

The next thing you need to do is to make good sleep a priority just like other healthy habits that you have. Take note of these points to help you sleep better:

- ✓ **Noise -** Make sure that your bedroom is extremely quiet; alternatively, you can use a white noise generator like a fan.
- ✓ **Be consistent -** Ensure that you maintain a relatively consistent bedtime and wake time. You can easily disrupt your routine during the week by staying up late and sleeping in on weekends.
- ✓ **Create a bedtime routine -** You need to come up with some bedtime routine or rituals that are relaxing and familiar. Avoid all electronic gadgets when it's time to sleep because things like movies, smartphones, television, computer, and others can disrupt sleep.
- ✓ **Avoid stimulants -** You should stay away from stimulants such as caffeine even during the day. Avoid taking nicotine as well as other stimulants because they affect the quality of sleep.

✓ Endeavor to get 30 minutes of sun exposure each day - preferably with exercise.

✓ **Temperature -** The temperature in your bedroom needs to be slightly cool; between 66-72 F or 18-22 C.

✓ **Exercise -** Exercise is one of the things you can do to enhance sleep, but it's not always advisable to exercise close to your sleep time.

✓ Don't eat large meals less than four hours before bed

Always bear in mind that sleep has no substitute, so you need to deliberately improve the quality and quantity of sleep you get every day. This will, in turn, help you enjoy the health benefits of eating good and nutritious diets.

# Final Thoughts

Living a healthy and successful life is not by chance, especially with the increase in the availability of unhealthy food and lifestyle choices. Nowadays, it's becoming increasingly difficult to make the right choices in the foods we eat and the things we drink. This has increased the number of obese people in various cities around the world. It even gets worse with the increase in the number of conflicting information regarding what we should eat and the ones we shouldn't eat.

What this book has succeeded in doing is to as much as possible, eliminate the difficult and confusing information regarding nutrition and diet and make it easy for you to live a healthy life without being overwhelmed. Eating healthy foods and living a healthy lifestyle is undoubtedly the best way to enjoy good health and a fulfilled life. I hope you enjoyed reading this book and remember; what differentiates successful people from unsuccessful people is action. Take action now, and enjoy a healthy life.

# Sources


Aetna. (2016). Do you know how much salt and sugar you consume every day? Retrieved on August 28, 2019 from https://news.aetna.com/2016/05/know-much-salt-sugar-consume-every-day/

Andrews, R. (n.d). All About Sleep. Retrieved on August 28, 2019 from https://www.precisionnutrition.com/all-about-sleep

Caffelle, J. (2019). Why Fruits and Vegetables Are Important. Retrieved on August 28, 2019 from https://www.familyeducation.com/life/general-nutrition/why-fruits-vegetables-are-important

Ferriera, M. (2018). 6 Essential Nutrients and Why Your Body Needs Them. Retrieved on August 26, 2019 from https://www.healthline.com/health/food-nutrition/six-essential-nutrients

Harvard Health Publishing. (2009). 13 ways to add fruits and vegetables to your diet. Retrieved on August 28, 2019 from https://www.health.harvard.edu/staying-healthy/13-ways-to-add-fruits-and-vegetables-to-your-diet

Harvard T. H Chan. (n.d). The Nutrition Source: Vegetables and Fruits. Retrieved on August 28, 2019 from https://www.hsph.harvard.edu/nutritionsource/what-should-you-eat/vegetables-and-fruits/

Healthy Living. (2017). How to Eat More Fruit and Vegetables. Retrieved on August 28, 2019 from https://www.heart.org/en/healthy-living/healthy-eating/add-color/how-to-eat-more-fruits-and-vegetables

Hughes, L. (2017). How Does Too Much Sugar Affect Your Body? Retrieved on August 28, 2019 from https://www.webmd.com/diabetes/features/how-sugar-affects-your-body

James, L. (2017). Sleep Is as Important as Diet and Exercise. Retrieved on August 28, 2019 from https://extension.psu.edu/sleep-is-as-important-as-diet-and-exercise

Kubala, J. (2018). 11 Reasons Why Too Much Sugar Is Bad for You. Retrieved on August 28, 2019 from https://www.healthline.com/nutrition/too-much-sugar#section1

Laskey, J. (2015). The Health Benefits of Water. Retrieved on August 27, 2019 from https://www.everydayhealth.com/water-health/water-body-health.aspx

Mentzer, A. P. (2019). How Can I Tell When My Body Is Hydrated? Retrieved on August 28, 2019 from https://www.livestrong.com/article/438381-how-can-i-tell-when-my-body-is-hydrated/

Miller, S. G. (2016). How to Eat Healthy (and Cut Sugar, Salt and Fat). Retrieved on August 28, 2019 from https://www.livescience.com/57290-eat-healthy-this-year.html

Robinson, L., Segal, J., and Segal, R. (2019). Organic Foods: What You Need to Know. Retrieved on August 28, 2019 from https://www.helpguide.org/articles/healthy-eating/organic-foods.htm

Silver, N. (2019). Why Is Water Important? 16 Reasons to Drink Up. Retrieved on August 27, 2019, from https://www.healthline.com/health/food-nutrition/why-is-water-important

Shannon, K. (n.d). Organic vs. Natural vs. GMO Foods and What You Need to Know About Each. Retrieved on August 28, 2019 from https://www.yogiapproved.com/health-wellness/organic-vs-natural-vs-gmo/

St. Pierre, B. (n.d). All About Eating Slowly. Retrieved on August 27, 2019 from https://www.precisionnutrition.com/all-about-slow-eating

Vancura, C. (2018). Drink up! Tips for staying hydrated. Retrieved on August 28, 2019 from https://www.centracare.com/blog/2018/january/drink-up-tips-for-staying-hydrated/